PACIFIER DILEMMA

BENEFITS, RISKS, AND BEST PRACTICES FOR YOUR CHILD

DR ANCHAL SHARMA

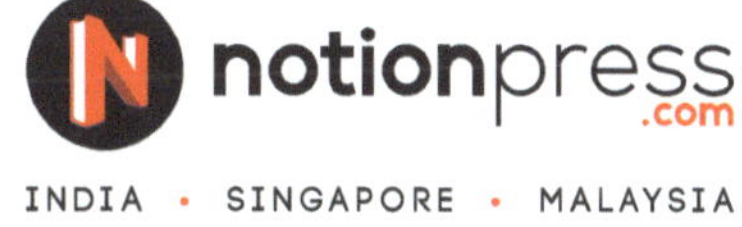

notionpress.com

INDIA · SINGAPORE · MALAYSIA

ISBN 979-8-89744-219-5

Pacifiers have proven to be the most debatable tool in infant care, praised for their soothing effects yet scrutinized for potential risks.

This book explores the benefits, risks, and best practices for using pacifiers to support a child's health and development. By examining scientific research, expert recommendations, and practical insights, this guide helps parents make informed choices. Whether you are considering introducing a pacifier or managing its use, this book provides clear, balanced advice to ensure it serves as a helpful tool rather than a source of concern.

ACKNOWLEDGMENTS

Writing this book would not have been possible without the support, guidance, and encouragement of my teachers. A heartfelt thank you to the parents and caregivers who shared their experiences, challenges, and successes helping to shape a practical and balanced perspective on pacifier use.

To my family and friends, your unwavering encouragement and patience have been invaluable throughout this journey. Your belief in the importance of this topic has kept me motivated.

Lastly, to the countless children whose comfort and well-being inspire this work. This book is dedicated to all my young patients.

CONTENTS

Chapter - 1

INTRODUCTION

Every parent's biggest concern for his child who loves sucking on a pacifier is "Will it affect his Dental Development?"

Children are born with adaptive reflexes (searching, sucking, and swallowing). Sucking begins between the 17th and 24th week of intrauterine life. Hence babies are often observed sucking their fingers inside their mother's uterus.[1]

The Physiological need for nutrition in a child is believed to initiate the Sucking behaviors. Current understanding of child development suggests that sucking behaviors also arise and continue due to psychological needs. The need for sucking can be satisfied through nutritive sucking, including breast and bottle feeding, or non-nutritive sucking on objects such as digits, pacifiers, and toys. The word Pacifier demonstrates its usefulness since it originates from the verb "to pacify" which means to calm down.

Pacifiers, also known as soothers, dummies, or artificial teats, facilitate non-nutritive sucking. While sucking behaviors are normal in infants and young children, prolonged duration of such behaviors may have consequences in regards to the developing oro- facial structures and occlusion.[2]

Since birth, infants have an instinct or urge that is considered to be the first feeding reflex established. This is essential for infants' survival, since it allows them to nurse and cling to their mothers, if the sucking urge is not completely satisfied by breast or bottle feeding the infant will have a surplus sucking urge which may either lead to frustration or engaging himself in non-nutritive sucking habits. Therefore, sucking not only has nutritional significance but also is a tremendous source of pleasure, self-gratification, comfort and relaxation.[3]

The habit of sucking is a reflex occurring in the oral stage of development and disappears during normal growth between the ages of 1 and 3 ½ years. It is the first coordinated muscular activity of the infant

Whereas, Non-nutritive sucking is the earliest sucking habit adopted by infants in response to frustration and to satisfy their urge and need for contact. Infants have used non-nutritive sucking with pacifiers in various forms for a very long time. It can soothe infants and young children, eliminate teething discomfort, and provide comfort during stressful episodes. Children who neither receive unrestricted breastfeeding nor have access to a pacifier may satisfy their need with alternative habits such as finger-sucking or sucking of other objects (a blanket or toy), which might be detrimental to their dentofacial development.[4]

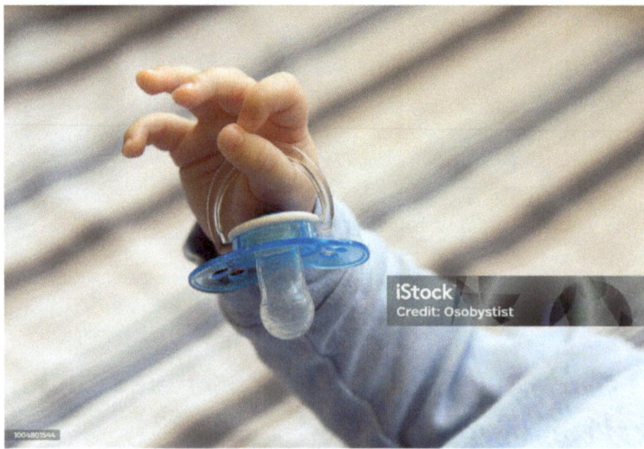

In some countries, as many as 90 percent of all children develop an initial sucking habit (Zadik et al. 1977, Modeer et al. 1982, Larsson 1983). About half of those who start a finger-sucking habit still do so at 7 years of age (Larsson 1971, 1985).[5]

The newborn child exhibits a completely developed circumoral and intraoral muscular activity. Especially noticeable is the infant's tongue activity, which is manifested primarily in attempts to swallow and suck. During the first days of life apart from sucking at mealtimes, the child attempts to suck his fingers or a dummy, if available. However, a sucking habit cannot be considered established, until it has continued for some time. [6]

The infant has a sucking instinct that varies in degree among individuals but is usually powerful. After the child has taken the first cereal or mother's milk, a surplus sucking urge often remains. The extent of this surplus depends on the extent of the original urge and how much of it has been spent on nourishment intake. The surplus-sucking urge may be either frustrated or re-directed. For the child, the most attractive method is unrestricted non-nutritive sucking. If this possibility is not available, the child might choose between dummy and finger sucking to obtain satisfaction.[7]

Chapter – 2

HISTORY

Pacifiers have been around for a very long time. Small clay pacifiers have been found in Cypriot graves dating back to about 1000 BC, and breast-shaped pottery nipples have been recovered from Roman graves dating from around AD 100. Excavations of 3,000-year-old baby's tombs revealed objects made of clay in the shape of pigs, frogs, or horses with one hole where honey could be poured in and another hole, in the animal's mouth, that enabled the child to suck their content.[8]

Pacifiers' history dates back to 1000 years when they were first mentioned in the medical literature at the end of the 15th century by Metlinger (1473) and Rosslin (1513).[9]

However, in the early 1900s, pacifier use was condemned by the infant welfare movement. Various reformers referred to the pacifier as a product of "perverted American ingenuity", an "instrument of torture," and a "curse of babyhood." Clinicians and public health practitioners have raised concerns that the pacifier causes "nipple confusion" and thereby leads to early weaning. Avoidance of pacifiers constitutes step 9 of the World Health Organization.[7]

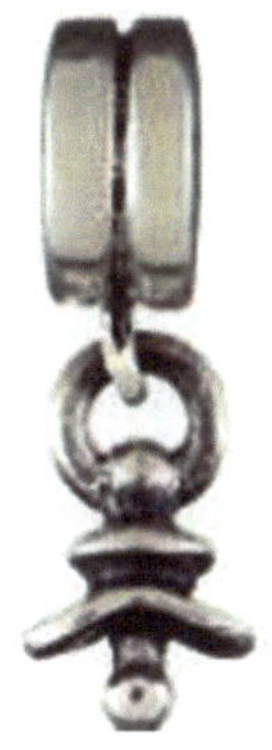
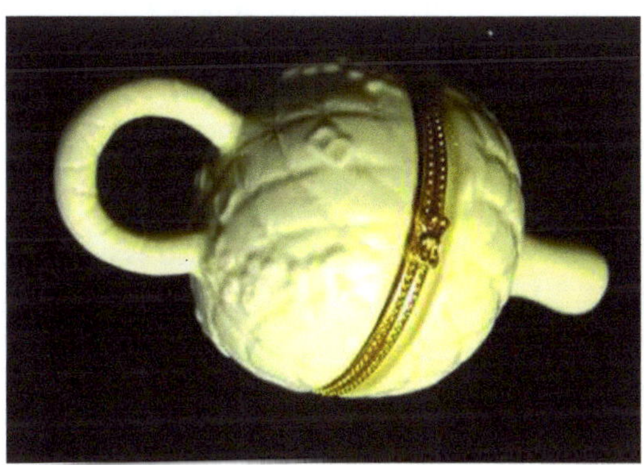
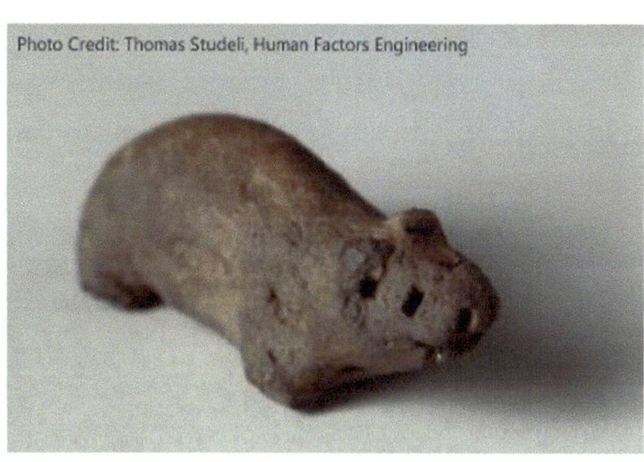

Ancient pacifiers were made from rags or chamois into which bread crumbs and sugar were placed and then tied in the shape of a nipple. Whenever the child cries, these are moistened and introduced into his or her mouth.[7]

Pacifiers used to be large enough so that children could not swallow it, and to its one end was a ring that could be fastened to a baby's clothes or crib.[8]

Chapter – 3

INCIDENCE AND PREVALENCE

Early descriptions of sucking appeared in the literature as early as the fifteenth and sixteenth centuries. The prevalence of the habit, as well as its etiology, possible consequences, and treatment were widely studied. There is a controversy concerning the etiology and treatment of the habit. One school of thought considers the habit as a normal development phenomenon that states no interference is necessary. Ravn suggests that one should not interfere with the habit, as usually it stops by itself and any intervention may cause unexpected and unfavorable side effects and complications.[10]

The other school of thought associates this habit with open-bite, posterior cross-bite, exaggerated overjet and overbite, temporomandibular joint problems, diastema, retrusive mandible position, and tongue and lip posture changes.

Baalack and Frisk suggested 7 years as a critical age for stopping the habit. They also state that dam ages from sucking a pacifier are less extensive than those caused by thumb -sucking. The extent of the damage also depends upon the habit's duration, and frequency.[11]

Prolonged dummy or finger–sucking habit is taken as one which prevails until at least 6 – 7 years of age. Children with a prolonged dummy–sucking habit are reported rarely. Many authors believe that prolonged sucking habits are due to emotional disturbances.

Andersson and Tode (1971) stated that a sucking habit in an older child is a sign of disharmony and may even be regarded as a psychological problem. According to Freud, the child has to pass through certain phases during its mental development; for example, the oral, anal, and genital phases. A requirement for successful emotional development is that each one of these phases must be completed and discontinued before the child enters the following phase. The sucking urge is, according to Freud, an urge which had to be satisfied during the oral phase. On the other hand, if the sucking habit continues into the next phase of the child's emotional development, a fixation on the habit will arise. Another possible explanation of a prolonged sucking habit is, according to this theory, that the child breaks the sucking habit at the end of the oral phase, and then, as a result of some sort of psychological stress, restarts the sucking habit some years later. This is called regression. Both fixation and regression are considered to be symptoms of mental disturbances. It is maintained that forced cessation of a sucking habit may mean that the mental disturbance is manifest in some other way such as enureses.[12]

Most children are able to stop sucking their fingers on their own. However, if this habit continues once their permanent teeth begin to emerge, it's important to encourage the child to stop. Scolding or punishing the child may discourage them and have negative effects. Instead, other strategies can be more effective. For example, praising the child and offering rewards for not sucking their fingers can help them feel a sense of accomplishment and increase their motivation to stop. If the child tends to suck their finger during idle moments, it may be helpful to distract them with activities or fun. Additionally, it can be beneficial to explain, in a way the child can understand, why they should stop finger-sucking.[13]

At the international symposia held in Brussels (1986) and in Chicago (1988), researchers concluded that there appears to be an increase in non–nutritive sucking in children in industrialized countries, possibly due to changes in parental responsibilities and attitudes because of social and economic pressures. Development of commercially available devices has increased, and every year, several "newly" designed pacifiers of "dummies" are promoted to parents for consideration. Differences in parenting, social and economic pressures also greatly influence the frequency and duration of non–nutritive sucking.[14]

Many reports from the literature and clinical observations by practitioners and investigators have also suggested that prolonged non–nutritive sucking may lead to dentofacial deformities. The effects of non–nutritive sucking on dentofacial development can be investigated by observing and measuring various skeletal and dental relationships. Clinical investigations report skeletal and dental changes, which involve proclination of the maxillary incisor.

Larsson and Lindsten reported that Swedish children with a sucking habit at three years of age had a prevalence of posterior cross-bites of 21%, while only 5% of the non–sucking children had cross-bites. Inter-canine measurements also showed that in dummy and finger–suckers, the maxillary width was narrower compared with that in the non–suckers, with a tendency for broader mandibular jaws in some dummy–sucking groups.

Lindner (Sweden), in a longitudinal study of four-year-olds with sucking habits, has demonstrated that the maxillary transverse measurements steadily decreased if the habit persisted, with a pronounced increase in posterior cross-bites in children with a persistent habit after age two.[14]

At the international symposia held in Brussels (1986) and in Chicago (1988), researchers concluded that;

1. The prevalence of sucking habits is increasing in industrialized countries.

2. With continuous non–nutritive sucking, there is increase in maxillary transverse width and posterior cross-bites in the primary dentition.

3. Children who are given pacifiers discontinue habit earlier than children who suck their finger thumbs.

4. Early prevention and correction of posterior cross-bite is recommended, especially where there is mandibular shift and asymmetry of the midline.

5. Ultrasound and EMG may be useful for studies on sucking disorders.

6. There is a need for collaborative studies with psychologists, sociologists, and allied health professionals to understand better the effects of parental practices, social and economic pressures, and section of diets on nutritive and non–nutritive sucking habits.

Data have also shown a slight increase in breastfeeding. It is more prevalent in developed environments, more common in towns than in villages, and among educated mothers than among the unschooled. The current prevalence of non-nutritive sucking habits at various ages has been reported between 61 and 95%, and Larsson states that pacifier users are in the majority in Scandinavia.[15]

Pacifier use has been associated with malocclusions in all three planes of spaces. Anterior open bites have been reported in as many as 74%. Posterior crossbites have been described in pacifier users as young as 24 months, while others have described a prevalence of 5 to 19%. Increased overjet (^{3} 4mm) has been noted in 17 to 79% of pacifier users. An increased prevalence of Class II canines and distal step primary molars also has been reported.[14]

Compared to habit free children, children with a history of pacifier use have a significantly higher occurrence of increased overjet a greater mean overjet, and reduced overbite. The prevalence of posterior crossbites and open–bites were also higher among children with a habit history.

The effect of prolonged sucking on dentofacial development has been controversial. Even more contentious is its prevention or the time when it is appropriate to intervene and stop the habit, More extensive studies are required in this field.

Chapter – 4

FEEDING AND DENTOFACIAL DEVELOPMENT

At the end of the pre-industrial era, as the habit of breastfeeding became less frequent, nonnutritive sucking (NNS) habits became more frequent. Until then, breastfeeding on demand was the predominant method of feeding infants. Breast sucking fulfilled both the infants' nutritional and emotional needs.[16]

Although studies show no significant differences in the number of malocclusions between breastfed and non-breastfed children, it has been found that breastfeeding encourages correct intermaxillary relationships.

Gedicke in his study claims that forward movements of the mandible occurred more quickly in breastfed infants than in bottle-fed infants. However, In a study by Heckmann et al a difference in the frequency of Class II malocclusion between the two groups is not confirmed.[17]

According to Hummel et al, growth of the child's oral structures is influenced by the oral part of the nipple and pacifier, while Meyers et al does not mention any possible relationship between nipple usage and the need for orthodontic treatment.[17,18]

In studying the etiology of dental crowding, Dandoit especially emphasized the substitution of bottle feeding for breast feeding as an important factor. The way an infant feed plays some role in the occurrence of diastemas between the anterior primary teeth. There were no statistically significant relationships between the prevalence of overjet and overbite and the way the child was fed. As far as its (breast–feeding) influence on the growth of the stomatognathic system is concerned, the conclusions are slightly more complex. Numerous endogenous and exogenous factors influence the occurrence of malocclusion.[17,18]

Therefore, it is important to recognize the influence of unfavorable factors on the growth and development of the oral and facial structures and the influence of favorable factors, such as breast feeding.[17]

Yarrow (1954), Graber (1963), and Najera (1963) believe that bottle feeding significantly influences a child's acquisition of digital habits. They generally observed that breast-fed infants have the lowest prevalence of digital habits. On the other hand, Klackenberg (1949, 1971), Traisman and Traisman (1958), and Porter (1964) concluded that the method of feeding had no appreciable influence on the acquisition of digital habits.[19]

Larsson (1985) indicated that in the last 15 years there has been a decrease in the number of children with a finger sucking habit and an increase in the number of dummy suckers. Larsson (1986) in a later review explained that continuous dummy sucking in the primary dentition usually is associated with an anterior open bite and an increased prevalence of posterior crossbite.[20]

Klackenberg (1949) and Popovich and Thompson (1973) believed that the use of a pacifier for non–nutritive sucking decreases the prevalence of the infant's acquiring a digit sucking habit. Popovich and Thompson (1973) concluded that since digital habits increase the prevalence of malocclusion, infants should be encouraged to use a pacifier as a prophylactic measure.[21,32]

Although each specialty (Pediatrician, Pediatric dentist and orthodontist) might be interested in various aspect of child development, collectively their objective is to ensure that the infant is provided with: 1) good nutrition, 2) optimal physical growth, 3) optimal emotional growth, and 4) optimal dental and facial growth. Hence it is important to be cautious while using pacifier for a child as it promotes early weaning depriving the child of the various benefits, he may gain from breast feeding.

Chapter – 5

THERAPEUTIC EFFECTS/ANALGESIC EFFECTS OF SWEET SOLUTIONS AND PACIFIERS

Ancient literature mentions that pacifiers immersed in alcoholic beverages (brandy) or containing opiates, were being used to calm down those children who were hungry or feeling pain, "making them fall asleep."[16]

Pacifiers and sugar solutions given unnecessarily to healthy neonates are not proven to be "simple and safe interventions". World Health Organization recommends exclusive breastfeeding, no food or drink other than breast milk, unless medically indicated should be given. Anything that may interfere with the establishment of lactation or undermine the mother's confidence in breast feeding is to be avoided. [22]

Treating pain in the newborn is essential firstly, for ethical reasons, and secondly, because pain can lead to decreased oxygenation, haemodynamic instability, or increased intracranial pressure. Recent research has shown that even short term pain can have lasting negative effect. This knowledge has led many neonatal teams to develop strategies to alleviate pain caused by diagnostic and therapeutic procedures undergone by newborns.

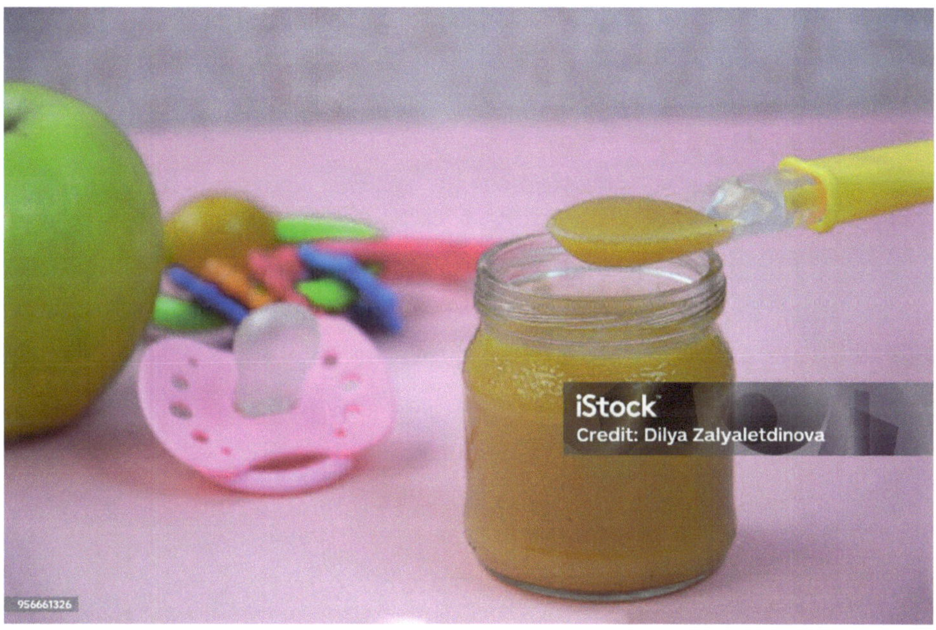

The analgesic effects of concentrated sucrose and glucose and pacifiers are clinically apparent in newborns, pacifiers being more effective than sweet solutions. The association of sucrose and pacifier showed a trend towards lower scores compared with pacifiers alone. These simple and safe interventions should be widely used for minor procedures in neonates.

Multiple studies state that the use of NNS relieves stress during painful procedures in newborns and infants, both when used alone and in combination of sugary solutions and music therapy. Although use of pacifier may modify responses measured on rating scale. Analgesic effects of both pacifiers and sweet solutions are clinically apparent and that pacifiers are more effective than sweet solutions alone. Non-nutritive sucking on a pacifier was more successful in producing analgesia in neonates during venepuncture than the use of glucose or sucrose solutions.

Cambell et al conducted a study based on the scale *douleur aigue dunouveau-ne*, This scale uses facial expression, limb movements, and vocal expression to give a score between 0 and 10. Low scores mean no or little pain, and higher scores mean that the infant experiences more pain. The study concluded that the groups whose treatment included a pacifier have a lower mean score and show a less varied response to the stimulus of venipuncture. [23]

Although Carbajal et al suggested that the less varied response to the stimulus is due to the pacifier itself. The ability to express a range of facial expressions will be modified by sucking on a pacifier in a way that reduces the possible responses on the rating scale. It would be interesting to see infant ratings without venipuncture on the rating scale with and without pacifiers.[24]

It has also been reported that oral sucrose administered via a nipple is effective for pain relief in neonatal circumcision. This analgesic effect may be more due to the pacifier than sucrose.

"Sweet flavoured pacifiers can calm a crying baby but should never be regarded as providing major analgesia". Likewise, measurement of the endocrine response alone is inadequate. An example is that pacifiers reduce the behavioral response to pain but do not reduce the endocrine response.[23]

Although sweet solutions are effective in reducing pain in newborns they cannot be considered as perfect analgesics. The precise mechanism by which pacifiers relieve pain remains to be identified. It has been suggested that two processes may play a part. The first is sensory dominance; as sucking is a powerful source of perceptual information for infants the sensations it elicits may have priority in the deployment of attentional resources and thus effectively mute pain. The second hypothesis is that pacifiers reduce infant response to pain by facilitating self-regulation. The provision of pacifiers enhances infants' ability to regulate their response to pain by allowing sucking. Elicitation of sucking with a pacifier enables infants to control one source of incoming stimuli - oral stimulation – through their activity.[24]

Chapter – 6

HARMFUL EFFECTS

Humans have used nonnutritive sucking (NNS) with pacifiers in various forms for possibly thousands of years. NNS can soothe infants and young children, assist with transitioning to sleep, alleviate teething discomfort, and provide comfort during stressful episodes. The use of pacifiers has been a topic of discussion since 1970, its use has been contraindicated not only because it causes nipple confusion but also because it postpones breastfeeding leading to an early weaning.

The dental literature has also focused on the changes pacifiers create on the occlusion and period tissues. While many studies have shown the benefits of pacifier use, such as a decrease in the possibility of sudden infant death syndrome (SIDS) and adjunctive pain relief explaining its widespread use worldwide, others stress its shortcomings. Pacifier use is debatable as it is also associated with several health issues.

Long-term nonnutritive sucking habits may lead to occlusal abnormalities, including open bite and posterior cross-bite. While continuous nonnutritive sucking habits of 48 months or longer produce the greatest changes in dental arch and occlusal characteristics, children with shorter sucking durations also had detectable differences from those with minimal habit durations.[25]

A peculiar distribution and variable decay severity in different teeth in the same child has been observed. The maxillary incisors were severely decayed and the mandibular incisors were unscathed. This can be attributed to the fact that during sucking, the natural or artificial nipple rests against the palate, .while the tongue lies over the lower teeth. Liquid from the mother's breast or nursing bottle may bathe all of the teeth except the lower incisors, which are physically protected by the tongue. If the child dozes with the nipple in its mouth, the liquid will pool against the upper incisors. If the liquid contains a fermentable carbohydrate, it will be acted upon by the oral bacteria resulting in the production of the acids that dissolve the teeth. Thus the upper incisors are most ravaged while the lower incisors are protected by the tongue and salvia from the mandibular salivary glands.[26]

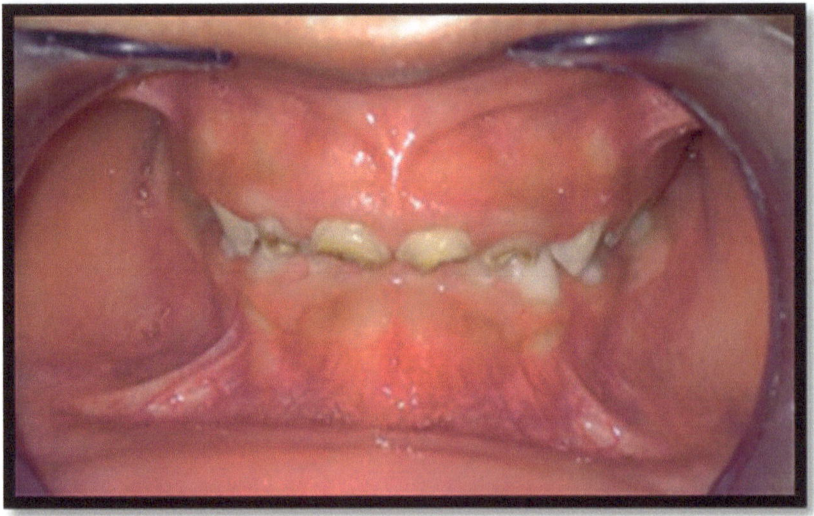

Figure: Early Childhood caries in a child

Nonnutritive sucking can be just as damaging to the teeth when a pacifier is sweetened with a decay-promoting agent. A favorite of mothers, especially in England and Germany, is the use of a honey-dipped pacifier since the baby is born. The writer has seen two American children of German ancestry who were allowed to suck a honey-sweetened pacifier. The results to the children's teeth were the same as already described in which the upper incisors were decayed to the gum line while the lower incisors remained unaffected.[26]

Pacifiers and otitis media :

Otitis media is a common childhood infectious disease, second only to the common cold, characterized by middle ear inflammation. It is a recurrent disease that, if untreated, can progress from the acute stage, lasting up to 3 weeks, to the sub-acute states, lasting between 3 weeks and 3 months, and the chronic stage, lastings for more than 3 months.

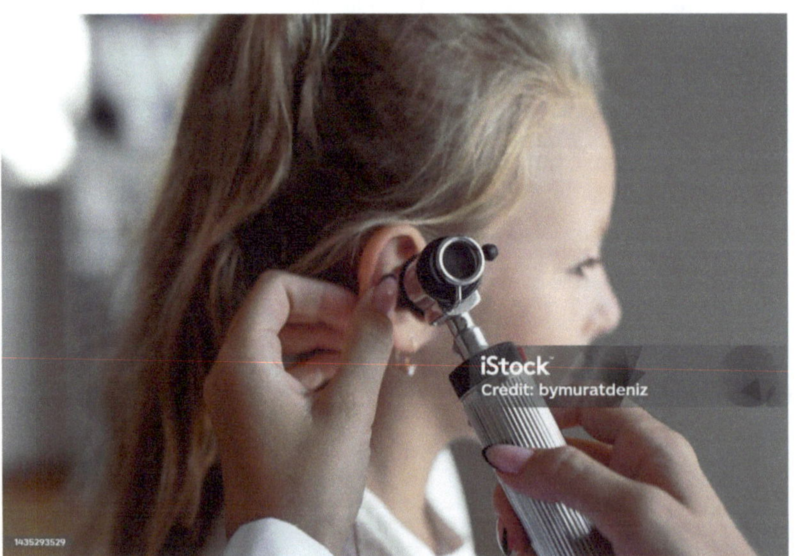

Although studies have shown that pacifier use is a risk factor for otitis media and malocclusion, the reasons for this are unknown. A possible explanation for an increase in cases of otitis media with pacifier use is that the pacifier could elevate the soft palate and impair the normal functions of the eustachain tube. An abnormally patent eustachian tube could result in a reflux of nasopharyngeal secretions into the tube, enhancing development of otitis media.

Lubianca Neto et al found that pacifiers are a risk factor for the development of recurrent acute otitis media. Niemela et al observed that those children who used pacifier had a higher risk of having recurrent acute otitis media in comparison with those who did not have this habit.[27] Also, the pacifiers could spread microorganisms when used in small, close contact areas like day care centers. 80% of positive cultures were found in a study with Staphylococcus and Candida being the most frequent genera of germs.[28]

Another study conducted by Mattos-Graner et al in Brazil found funguses in the mouth of 58.3% of children who were between 0-8 months of age and provided with a history of pacifier use.[29]

Traumatic Gingival Recession In Infants:

The habit of dummy sucking is widely recognized as a cause of malocclusion in young children. In addition, when the dummy is used as a vehicle for any one of a large number of sugary substances, it is associated with a specific type of rampant caries which first attacks the labial surfaces of the upper incisors.

Some children, who suck dummies, do so in unconventional ways. One of these ways is illustrated where the infant's lower lip embraces a segment of the plastic shield, between the inner surface of the incisors and on the gums. If held in this position, the edge of the shield, during sucking, moves with an abrasive action and thus leads to gingival injury, recession and local loss of a alveolar bone. Majority of the children who practice this particular variation of the habit also exhibit in addition to gingival recession, other features that are more commonly associated with dummy sucking.

Injury to gum and alveolar bone is commonly seen, although it may not be a cause of concern, as the gingival contour will normally become reestablished with the eruption of the permanent incisors. However, an injury having an almost identical clinical appearance may be seen in a small number of children, who for obscure and complex reasons injure their gums, usually with their finger nails. If the injuries are of the latter origin, the implications are more serious, and therefore the clinician must establish with certainty the cause of this type of recession when it occurs.[30]

The influence of a pacifier on infant's arousals from sleep:

The risk of sudden infant death during sleep was postulated to decrease with the use of a pacifier and by conditions facilitating arousal from sleep.[31]

Infants using pacifiers during sleep had lower auditory arousal thresholds than those who did not use a pacifier during sleep. Pacifier sucking was shown to favor higher blood oxygen saturation values and total sleep time. It was speculated that the use of a pacifier prevents the tongue from sealing off the airways, reduces the frequency and duration of gastroesophageal refluxes, decreases the prevalence of prone sleeping, favors mouth breathing, and increases respiratory drive and sensory inputs in muscles responsible for the patency of the upper airway because arousals from sleep were also hypothesized to protect an infant against sudden death during sleep.

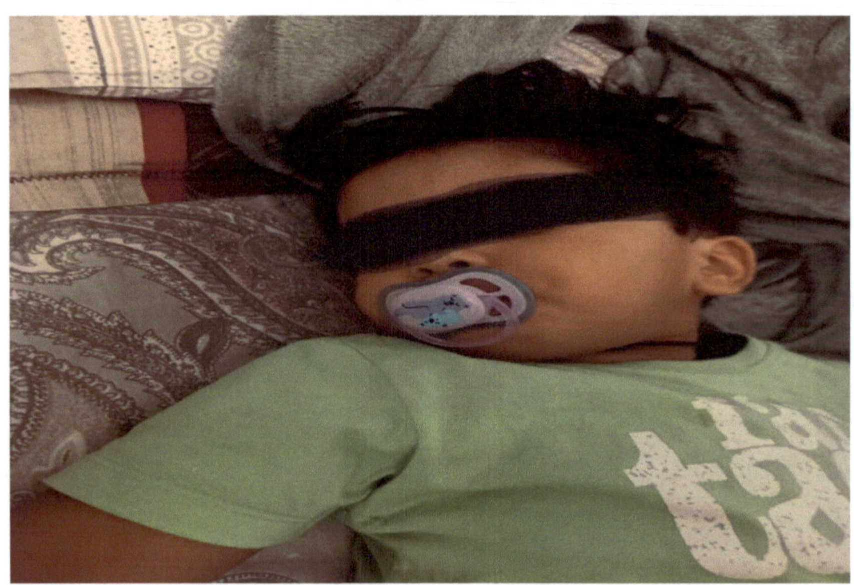

Figure: A child using a Pacifier during sleep

However, significantly fewer auditory stimuli were required to induce polygraphic arousals in healthy infants who usually slept with a pacifier than in infants who did not use a pacifier. These findings could explain the reported association between the use of a pacifier and a low risk for sudden death during sleep as being the result of an enhanced arousal from sleep. Increases in auditory arousal thresholds were seen in conditions reported to increase the risk for sudden death during sleep such as prone sleep and prenatal exposure to cigarette smoke. [31]

Not much of explanation are given as to why, the use of a pacifier was associated with lower auditory arousal thresholds. Pacifier users and nonusers could not be differentiated by factors known to modify arousal thresholds such as time of the night, exposure to light, background noise levels, type of auditory stimulus, time of feeding, or environmental temperature. Our findings could be related to the disruptive effect of losing a pacifier during sleep, because most infants lost their pacifier after 30 minutes of continuous sleep. The loss of a pacifier was reported to favor infant's restlessness and frequent night walking.

Pacifier users were significantly more frequently bottle-fed than breastfed. Associations between pacifier use and fewer or shorter breast-feeding periods were reported. The breast-fed infants had a lower arousal threshold than the bottle-fed infants.[31] Not much of investigation for other factors such as, expiratory CO_2 levels or esophageal refluxes are done so far.

The relationship between pacifier use and sudden infant death syndrome:

Sudden infant death syndrome (SIDS) is defined as "the sudden death of the infant less than 1 year of age which remains unexplained after a thorough case investigation, including the performance of a complete autopsy, examination of the death scene, and review of the clinical history. Infant's sleeping environment as providing factors affecting the risk for SIDS. These include sleeping position, bedding, bed sharing, and breast or bottle-feeding. The peak incidence of the role of pacifier use in SIDS has been evaluated in several observational studies.

Mitchell et al were the first to publish data linking pacifier use with a protective effect against SIDS. In the case-control study, the reported usage rate of pacifiers with the last sleep of SIDS victims was about half of the reported for control infants at the sleep period chosen for comparison in their study.

Hauck et al. found that in studies where a variety of factors were controlled, 'usual' pacifier use was associated with an approximately 30% reduction in the risk of SIDS.[33]

The effect of pacifier use on breast-feeding :

A mother's decision to breastfeed her newborn infant is based on multiple factors. Recent times have witnessed a trend toward reductions in the initiation and duration of breast-feeding, particularly in developing countries. Several factors possibly associated with decreased breast-feeding are:

1. Lower maternal educational levels;
2. Lower socioeconomic status (SES);
3. First-born children;
4. Socio-cultural factors;
5. Maternal employment outside the home;
6. Marketing of infant formulas;
7. Influence of heath care personnel;
8. Insufficient milk syndrome, mastitis, or abnormalities of breast or nipple.

Pacifier use as a negative factor associated with breast-feeding received little attention until the 1990s. Early in that decade, the United Nations Children's Fund and the World Health Organization began a joint program in the Baby –Friendly Hospital Initiative (BFHI), a comprehensive effort to encourage health care providers to establish hospital programs to promote and support breast-feeding. The BFHI program recognizes rewards health care facilitates that adopt its recommendations and encourage breast-feeding. Step 9 of the program states: Give no artificial teats or pacifiers to breast-feeding infants. Schubiger et al, determined that bottle-feeding with or without pacifier use did not influence the duration of breast-feeding during the infants' first 6 months of life.[7]

Palatal deformations caused by pacifier:

According to a study conducted in Finland, pacifier use can deform infant's palates. These researchers conducted a study of 141 predominantly breast-fed infants to determine the effects pacifiers or finger-sucking had on the infants' developing palates and occlusion.

In the first 12 months of the study, they found that 76 percent of the children used a pacifier, 19 percent did not have any sucking habits, and 5 percent sucked their fingers. When the children were six months old, researchers found a depression resembling the shape of the pacifier nipple in the palatal tissues of 87 percent of the children who used pacifiers.

When the children were 12 months old, researchers found palatal tissues deformations in 96 percent of the pacifier using children. Among children who sucked their fingers, 71 percent had similar depressions, and only 29 percent of children who did not exhibit any sucking habits had deformations.

Researchers concluded that infant's palatal tissues are highly plastic and readily reflect the influences of sucking habits. In addition, they said it is probable that the duration and intensity of pacifier sucking, as well as the size and shape of the pacifier, all are factors that contribute to the extent of the deformation. Prolonged pacaifier use can also cause constricted palatal arch.

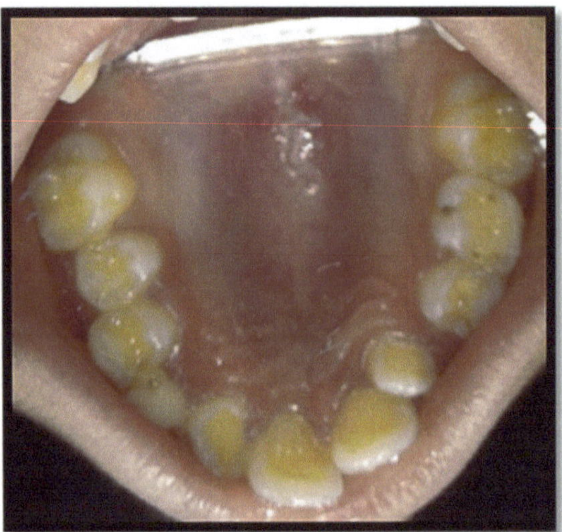
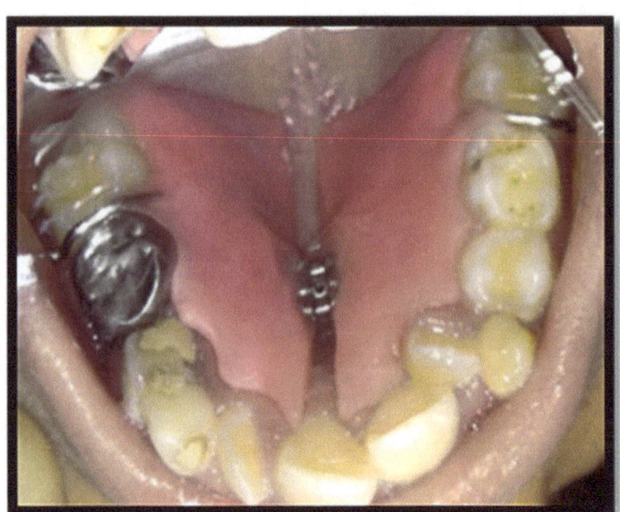

Figure: Treatment of constricted maxillary arch using expansion plate.

Researchers continue to study these children to determine if the deformations disappear after they stop using pacifiers. They will also study the long-term effects of pacifier use on the maxillary arch and occlusion.[34]

Pacifier and Dental Caries

The use of pacifiers has long since been associated with the occurrence of dental caries in kids.

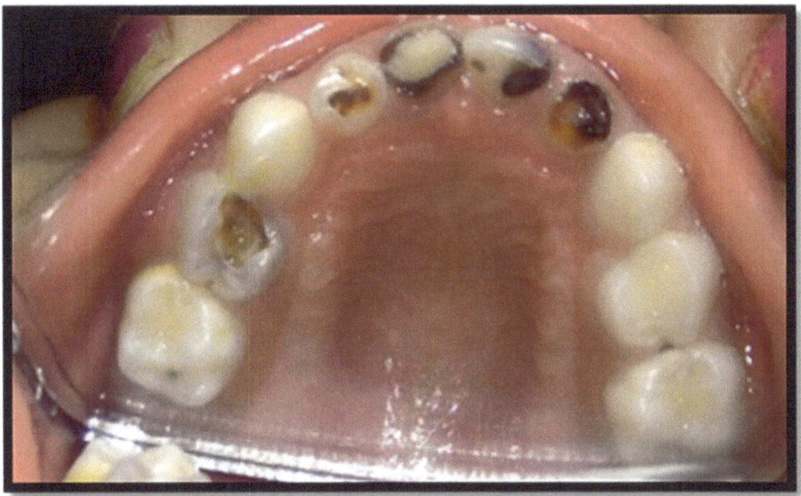

Figure: A 6-year-old child with multiple carious lesions and History of Pacifier use.

Yonezu & Yakushiji found that the use of pacifiers at 18 months of life is a risk factor for the development of caries[35]

Similarly, in a study by Vazquez- Nava et al the risk is twice as high in children who use pacifiers than in those without the habit.[36]

Effect of Pacifier on Speech

Sucking, chewing, swallowing, and breathing are vital reflexive functions for human beings. The stomatognathic system is responsible for nutrition, dental stability in its correct angles and preparation of phono articulatory organs adapting them for speech. Stimulation of these functions prevents communication disorders.

When used inappropriately, the pacifier harms speech development as it fills the oral cavity restricting the ability to babble, mimic sounds, and repeat words leading to impaired vocalization.[37]

Pacifiers have also been linked to being a risk factor for otitis relapse. Fluid inside the middle ear impairs hearing. Otitis is more frequent in the first year of life, and its relapse may cause speech development delay or problems.

Chapter – 7

ISSUES RELATED TO SAFETY OF PACIFIERS AND PACIFIER COMPONENTS

Pacifier safety issues can be of 3 types:

1) PHYSICAL

2) CHEMICAL AND

3) IMMUNOLOGICAL

Physical safety:

Pacifier materials and design, combined with improper usage, have contributed to reports of morbidity and mortality associated with mishaps. The following are reports regarding these incidents; Asphyxia has been reported several times over the past 30 years.[38]

Kravath described the asphyxiation of a 5 month old, who was using a pacifier that had a stylized mouse's head in place of the usual ring. Attempts to dislodge the pacifier from the pharynx by pulling on the mouse's had resulted in the nipple portion pulling through the flange. The flange remained in the pharynx, resulting in death.[39]

Simkiss et al described a more fortunate outcome in a 6 month old infant who began choking on her pacifier. The infant's parents were unable to remove it. A tracheostomy was performed in the emergency room, and the pacifier was eventually removed. The authors of both cases remarked on the force that was required to dislodge the pacifiers once the flanges were positioned behind the soft palate. Jones reported; an 8 month old who had swallowed a flanged pacifier with resultant respiratory distress, but the outcome was not fatal.[40]

Simkiss et al and Williams stated that ventilation holes in pacifier flange are essential. They also recommended that flange have minimum horizontal and vertical dimensions of 43 mm, and that manufacturers be required to place a ring behind the flange. [40,41]

A survey on strangulation reported cases in which cord attached to the pacifier caught on a part of the infant's crib. The authors noted that the United States Consumer Product Safety Commission (USCPSC) does not allow pacifiers to be sold with cord attached. Further, the USCPSC requires manufacturers to provide a warning with pacifier packaging that warns parents/ caregivers not to attach cords. The issue of the "grasp ring" is still a dilemma. Some suggest that they be banned because they are required to facilitate removal in case of aspiration.[42]

Izenberg et al reported an 18 month old infant, who strolled with a pacifier in her mouth, sufficed a laceration along the lower border of both alar cartilages. The lacerations were contiguous beneath the columella, the soft tissue covering the tip of the nose. The cause of this "cookie cutter" laceration was determined by noting the shape of the upper edge of the flange corresponded precisely to that of the laceration. [43]

Stubbs and Aburn reported on a 14 month old male who suffered a horizontal laceration below his right eye caused by his pacifier. The injury included a laceration of the conjunctiva and sclera, which led to extrusion of vitreous, discoloration of the iris, and sluggish reaction to light. Normal color and function returned after 1 week of treatment. [43]

Fenicia et al reported a case of infant botulism in a 9 week old female whose pacifier had been sweetened with honey contaminated with Clostridium botulinum spores. The authors recommended that honey be avoided as a sweetening agent in infant under the age of 1 year. A report by Pedra et al described 5 cases of large traumatic ulcers of 2 weeks to 4 months duration on the palates of infants. The authors determined the cause of the ulcers to be traumatic from the use of standard bottle nipples in all 5 cases and pacifiers in 4 of the cases. The ulcers resolved after nipple orifices were enlarged and feeding position was corrected in 3, pacifier use was discontinued in 1, and bottle and pacifier use was discontinued in another.[44]

The USCPSC promulgated pacifier safety standards in October 1976. These standards require that pacifiers be designed and constructed to protect the user under reasonably foreseeable conditions of use from pharyngeal obstruction, strangulation, wounding, or aspiration of the pacifier or any of its components. The regulations specify the size of the flange, the strength of the components, and means for testing to meet these standards. The USCPSC also forbids the sale of pacifiers with a cord, ribbon, chain or similar device attached, and it requires package warnings to caregivers to "never tie pacifiers or other items around your child's neck".

Chemical safety: N- nitrosamines in pacifiers:

During the processing of natural rubber and the creation of synthetic rubber products, a variety of substances are added including accelerators, antioxidants, reinforcing agents, N-nitrous compounds, and various amines and alkyl carbamates. N-nitrosamines and N-nitramines form when stabilizers and accelerators derived from dialkylamines contact the nitrosating agents. Despite repeated extractions of N-nitrosamines and their precursors, these compounds may persist for the lifetime of a manufactured rubber article. When they get in touch with saliva, these product volatize and may be harmful for health.[38]

Volatile N-nitrosamines have been shown in animal tests to be potent carcinogens. Studies have reported the presence of N-nitrosamines in baby bottle nipples and other rubber products, and have determined that these compounds can be extracted via an aqueous simulated saliva, suggesting that an infant could ingest them during feedings or NNS. Further, infants may also ingest N–nitrosamine precursors that may be nitrosated in the stomach combined with nitrite from the saliva. [45,46]

Concern over these compounds has prompted most counties to adopt regulations regarding baby nipples and pacifiers. In the United States, the regulations specify that no component of the pacifier may contain more than 20 parts per billion of total volatile N-nitrosamines as determined by dichloromethane extraction. Pacifiers may not have sharp points or edges painted with paint that contain more than 0.06% head.[47,48]

Immunologic safety; latex allergy:

The possibility of some children being allergic to latex came to light.

Makinen-Kiljunen et al reported allergies related to pacifier use in 3 infants. The conditions of all 3 improved when pacifier use was discontinued.[49]

Venuta et al reported a case of a child who used a pacifier and who developed a cough which was resistant to conventional treatment. Suspecting that the cough might have an allergic basis, the latex pacifier was replaced by silicone product. The cough abated, confirming the author's suspicions about latex allergy.[50]

Niggemann et al investigated the associations between early sensitization to latex and various lifestyle factors, including pacifier use. They enrolled almost 400 children from a prospective birth cohort study. by age 5 years, 20 (5%) demonstrated specific serum IgE to latex. Sensitization was evident after age 1, and 19 of the 20 sensitized children demonstrated increasing specific IgE levels over time. All 20 were atopic. The latex-allergic children had undergone significantly more operations than the non-allergic group. However, no differences were found between the latex-allergic and non-allergic children in exposure to pacifiers. The authors concluded that no risk factors for developing latex allergy could be identified in pacifier using children up to 5 years other than atopic predisposition and the number of surgical procedures.[51]

The USCPSC regulations do not address latex allergy, and no latex allergy warning is currently required on pacifier labels. Some silicone pacifiers, however, are labeled "non-latex" as a safety statement and, probably, a marketing tool. Parents and caregivers of children with latex allergies are quite aware of consumer products that contain latex and would likely be drawn to silicone products for their children.[38]

Recommendations:

A few rational steps can be taken to enhance the benefits and reduce the risks of pacifier use :

1) Educate parents and caregivers about the safe use of pacifiers.

2) Withhold the use of pacifiers until breast-feeding is established after that point; limit their use for soothing breast-fed infants.

3) Advise parents and caregivers to exercise judgment and restraint regarding pacifier use. They should be taught to avoid its use throughout the day.

4) Instruct parents and caregivers to clean pacifiers routinely and avoid sharing between siblings. Parents should not lick pacifiers to clean them. Parents should consider having several pacifiers to rotate through cycles of cleaning and use during the day.

5) Suggest to parents that pacifier use by curtailed beginning at 2 years of age and that pacifier habits be discontinued by or before age 4 to minimize the development of malocclusion.[18]

Chapter – 8

BEST PRACTICES FOR A CHILD WITH DUMMY SUCKING HABIT

Dummy and finger sucking habits are very common in the Western world. In some countries, as many as 90 % of children develop an initial sucking habit. It is more common today than it was 10 years ago and also persists for longer and often outdoors even when the child plays.

About half the children, who develop a finger–sucking habit, will still suck at 7 years of age. Most dummy-suckers have broken their habit by 3– 4 years of age. Therefore, the question of weaning the finger–suckers off the habit is more urgent than with dummy–sucking.

Although Dummy sucking normally stops at an acceptable age without any treatment the most common issue with dummy sucking is its incorrect placement by the child. About one-third of all dummy–suckers, for instance, suck their dummies with the shield partly inside the lower lip. This has detrimental effects on the dentition and even affects the thin marginal bone of the anterior part of the mandible. In rare cases, the asymmetric use of a dummy can have remarkable effects on the occlusion. The use of a dummy can aggravate a large median diastema.

Therefore, it is of utmost importance to prevent the child from using the dummy wrongly. Many of the problems described above can be controlled by educating the parents. Today many children suck their dummies almost full time.

It should be pointed out that dummy–sucking is a substitute for non–nutritive feeding or unrestricted breast-feeding and not a physiological part of the baby's growth, and should be used following this. The need for physical contact between mother and the baby should also be stressed.

Weaning a child off the pacifier early helps avoid dental issues, prevent speech delays, and encourage independence.

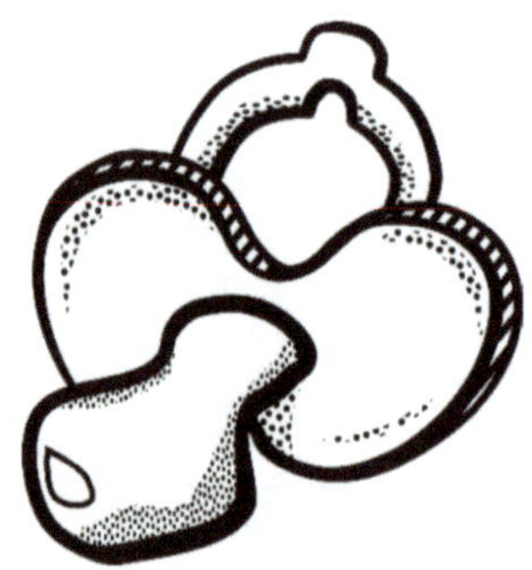

How to wean your baby off the pacifier (at 12-15 months old)

- Trying to eliminate the pacifier at times when the baby doesn't need to suck, try offering some other form of stimulation mobile, rattle or swinging chair. If teething seems to be the issue try offering a teether or cold wash cloth instead.

- If your baby protests and starts to cry, you could try to delay giving them their pacifier by distracting them with a toy or playing with them.

It's best to wean from the pacifier gently when the baby is content and distracted with other things. If you try to take it when they're already upset and your baby has a strong need to suck, withholding it may make them cry longer and get more upset. Also, it's worth noting that if you take the pacifier away at an age when the urge to suck for comfort is still strong, your baby may switch to sucking on something else like a thumb, or finger.

Once the baby is using pacifier only at night, introducing a comforting bedtime routine and a favorite toy or blanket can finally be weaned off the pacifier.

How to wean a toddler off the pacifier

The quick route

Explain to your toddler that in 3 days, you'll be taking away their pacifier because they're already big enough to manage without one. Repeat your message the following day.

On the day of reckoning, remove all pacifiers. The best practice is to offer your toddler another comfort toy like a teddy, blanket, whistle, or teether. Some parents like to use the story of a pacifier fairy, who comes to take the pacifiers in the house so other babies can use them, and leaves a new toy in its place.[52]

The slow route:

Slow and steady wins the race.

- **Toddler talk.** Talk to your toddler. Plant the idea that they can do it without a pacifier by telling them stories about other friends (real or imaginary) who did just that. Let your toddler see you bragging to their favourite teddy that very soon your toddler is going to put down their pacifier.

- **Share tools.** Show your child that they can manage without their pacifier by gently stretching out the time from when they ask for their pacifier and when you hand it over. Offer them other comfort measures instead. When they successfully go without the pacifier, praise them loudly.

- **Limit.** Use your instincts to figure out when your toddler really needs their pacifier and when they can go without it. Work towards setting times that the pacifier is used, for example, at nap time.

- **Give choices.** One of the best ways to work with toddler behaviour is to give acceptable choices. So with the pacifier, limit its use to certain places. The choice would be something like, "If you want your pacifier, it's in your room. Or, you can play out here without it. We can't use it here because that's not where the pacifier lives."

- **Reward.** Your child is venturing out of their comfort zone, and they deserve a reward for stretching. Some parents use sticker charts to help their child visualize how many days they've made it through without a pacifier. Some children respond better to other rewards. You know your child best.[52]

The AAPD (American Academy of Paediatric Dentistry) supports parents in the decision to introduce a pacifier based on their infant's needs and parental preferences, as it may be beneficial during the first few months of life in helping premature infants develop the sucking reflex.

AAPD stresses that educating parents on the risk of prolonged pacifier use after 12 months of age can increase the risk of acute otitis media, and beyond 18 months, it can affect the developing orofacial complex, leading to anterior open bite, posterior crossbite, and class II malocclusion.[53]

Important take-aways regarding pacifier use for Parents:

1. Wait before breastfeeding is well established before offering a pacifier to your baby.

2. Use a pacifier mainly for comfort and sleep and not as primary way to soothe the baby.

3. Choose the pacifier wisely. It is advisable to use a pacifier with a large shield to prevent your baby from putting the entire pacifier in their mouth.

4. Clean and sterilize the pacifier regularly to avoid infections spreading through germs.

5. Replace the pacifier every 2 months or when it shows signs of wear and tear.

6. Gradually wean your child off the pacifier around 18 months of age to minimize potential dental issues.

7. Never tie the pacifier around the baby's neck or hand.

Chapter - 9

CONCLUSION

The common belief passed down through generations is that pacifier calms down children, provide comfort, and make it a highly sort for object by parents.

Even though Health Professionals do not recommend its use, it has always found its way into the baby layette, Making its use a controversial topic.

Although pacifiers have been used to stimulate sucking in children with neuropathies, to coordinate sucking, swallowing, and breathing, and to reduce stress in painful procedures it is also associated with many harmful effects.

Pacifier use prevents babies from achieving breast sucking and induces an early weaning. It can cause allergies and increased risk of dental caries and infections which can also contribute to speech problems.

Eventually, the decision of whether to use or avoid the pacifier is for the family to make, and it is the responsibility of the health professionals to enlighten the family about the various pros and cons of pacifier use so that they can make an informed decision about it.

Chapter – 10

REFERENCES

1- S Diez, M Rocha. Pacifier habit: history and multidisciplinary view. J Pediatr (Rio J). 2009;85(6):480-489

2- Warren JJ, Levy SM, Nowak AJ, Tang MAS. Non-nutritive sucking behaviors in preschool children: a longitudinal study. Pediatr Dent 2000;22:187-191.

3- Zardetto CG del C, Rodrigues CRMD, Stefani FM. Effects of different pacifiers on the primary dentition and oral myofunctional structures of preschool children. Pediatr Dent 2002;24:552-560.

4- Turgeon-O'Brien H, Lachapella D, Gagnon PF, Larocque I, Maheu-Robert L. nutritive and nonnutritive sucking habits: A review. J Dent Child 1996;321-327.

5- Larsson E. Treatment of children with a prolonged dummy of finger-sucking habit. Eur J Orthodont1988;10:244-248.

6- Larsson EF, Dahlin KG. The prevalence and the etiology of the initial dummy-and finger-sucking habit. Am J Orthod 1985;87(5): 432-435.

7- Kramer MS, Barr RG, Dagenais S, Yang H, Jones P, Ciofani L et al. Pacifier use, early weaning, and cry / fuss behavior – a randomized controlled trial. JAMA 2001;28(3):322-326.

8- Baby-bottle museum. [website]. The history of the feeding bottle. http://www.babybottle-museum.co.uk/articles.html. Access: 17/01/2009.

9- Levin S. Dummies. S Afr Med J. 1971;45:237-240

10- JJ Ravn. The prevalence of finger and dummy sucking habit inCopenhagen children until the age of 3 years. Community Dent oral Epidemiology. 1974; 2(6):316-322

11- Zadik D, Stern N, Litner M. Thumb-and pacifier-sucking habits. Am J Orthod 1977;71(2):197-201.

12- Larsson E. The prevalence and etiology of prolonged dummy and finger-sucking habits. Eur J Orthodont1985;7:172-176.

13- American Academy of Pediatrics. Caring for your baby and young child. 5th ed. 2009. Pg-584, Birth to Age 5.

14- Nowak AJ. Feeding and dentofacial development. J Dent Res 1991;70(2) 159-160.

15- Larsson E. The influence of oral habits on the developing dentition and their treatment: clinical and historical perspectives. European journal of orthodontics. 2003; 26(3) 348-349

16- Fildes VA. Breasts, bottles, and babies: a history of infant feeding. Edinburgh University Press; 1986.

17- Bishara SE, Nowak AJ, Kohout FJ, Heckert A, Hogan MM. Influence of feeding and non-nutritive sucking methods on the development of the dental arches: longitudinal study of the first 18 months of life. Pediatr Dent 1987;9(1):13-21.

18- Juberg DR, Alfano K, Coughlin RJ, Thompson KM. An observational study of object mouthing behavior by young children. Pediatr2001;107:135142.

19- Najera A.Relationship between breast-feeding & bottle-feeding to craniofacial & dental development.2005;12:9-17

20- Larsson E. The effect of dummy-sucking on the occlusion: a review. Eur J Orthod. 1986;8:127-30.

21- Legovic M, Ostric L. The effects of feeding methods on the growth of the jaws in infants. J Dent Child 1991;253-255.

22- Vallena C, Savage F. Evidence for the ten steps to successful breast feeding.Geneva; World Health Organization.1998

23- Campbell c. Analgesic effects of sweet solutions and pacifier in term neonates. BMJ 2000; 320(7240):1002

24- Carbajal R, Chauvet X, Cougderc S, Olivier-Martin M. Randomized trial of analgesic effects of sucrose, glucose, and pacifiers in term neonates. BMJ 1993;319:1393-7.

25- Warren JJ, Bishara SE, Steinbock KL, Yonezu T, Nowak AJ. Effects of oral habits duration on dental characteristics in the primary dentition. JADA 2001;132:1685-1693

26- Ripa LW. Nursing habits and dental decay in infants : "Nursing bottle caries". J Dent Child 1978;274-275.

27- Lubianca Neto JF, Hemb L, Silva DB. Systematic literature review of modifiable risk factors for recurrent acute otitis media in childhood. J Pediatr (Rio J). 2006;82:87-96

28- Comina E, Marion K, Renaud FN, Dore J, Bergeron E, Freney J. Pacifiers: a microbial reservoir. Nurs Health Sci. 2006;8:216-23.

29- Mattos-Graner RO, de Moraes AB, Rontani RM, Birman EG. Relation of oral yeast infection in Brazilian infants and use of a pacifier. ASDC J Dent Child. 2001;68:33-36.

30- Stewart DJ, Kernohan DC. Traumatic gingival recession in infants – the result of a dummy sucking habit. Br Dent 1973;21:157-159.

31- Franco P, Scaillet S, Warmenbol V, Valente F, Groswasser J, Khan A. The influence of a pacifier on infants' arousals from sleep. J Pediatr2000;136:775-779.

32- Popovich F, Thompson T. thumb-and finger-sucking: its relation to malocclusion. Am J Orthod 1973;63(2):148-155.

33- Hauck FR, Omojokun OO, Siadaty MS. Do pacifiers reduce the risk of sudden infant death syndrome? A meta-analysis. Pediatrics. 2005;116:e716-23.

34- Palatal deformations caused by pacifiers. JADA 1999;130: 480-490

35- Yonezu T, Yakushiji M. Longitudinal study on influence of prolonged non-nutritive sucking habits on dental caries in Japanese children from 1.5 to 3 years of age. Bull Tokyo Dent Coll. 2008;49:59-63.

36- Vázquez-Nava F, Vázquez RE, Saldivar GA, Beltrán GF, Almeida AV, Vázquez RC. Allergic rhinitis, feeding and oral habits, toothbrushing and socioeconomic status. Effects on development of dental caries in primary dentition. Caries Res. 2008;42:141-147.

37- Shotts LL, McDaniel DM, Neeley RA. The impact of prolonged pacifier use on speech articulation: a preliminary investigation. CICSD. 2008;35:72-75.

38- Adair SM. Pacifier use in children : a review of recent literature. Pediatr Dent 2003;25:449-458.

39- Kravath RE. A lethal pacifier. Pediatrics. 1976; 58(6):853-855.

40- Simkiss DE, Sheppard I, Pal BR. Airway obstruction by a child's pacifier—could flange design be safer? Eur J Pediatr. 1998;157:252-254.

41- Williams MJ. The need for ventilation holes in children's pacifiers. Arch Emerg Med. 1991;8:59-62.

42- Feldman KW, Simms RJ. Strangulation in childhood: Epidemiology and clinical course. Pediatrics. 1980; 65:1079-1085.

43- Izenberg N, Izenberg P, Dowshen SA. Facial trauma from a rigid infant pacifier face shield. A patient re port and review of pacifier safety. Clin Pediatr. 1993;32:558-560.

44- Fenicia L, Ferrini AM, Aureli P, Pocecco M. A case of infant botulism associated with honey feeding in Italy. Eur J Epidemiol. 1993;9:671-673.

45- Ireland CB, Hytrek FP, Lasoski BA. Aqueous extraction of N-nitrosamines from elastomers. Am Ind Hyg Assoc J. 1980.41:859-900.

46- Preussmann R, Spiegelhalder B, Eisenbrand G. Re duction of human exposure to environmental N-nitroso compounds. Am Chem Soc Symp Ser. 1981;174:217-228.

47- Speigelhalder B, Preusmann R. Nitrosamines and rubber. In: H Bartsch, M Castegnaro, IK O'Neill, M Okada, eds. Nitroso compounds: occurrence, biological effects, and relevance to human cancer. IARC Scientific Publication No. 41. Lyon: IARC; 1982: 231-243.

48- Westin JB, Castegnaro MJ-J, Friesen MD. N-nitro samines and nitrosatable amines, potential precursors of N-nitramines, in children's pacifiers and baby bottle nipples. Environ Res. 1987;43:126-134.

49- Mäkinen–Kiljunen S, Sorva R, Juntunen–Backman K. Latex dummies as allergens. Lancet. 1992;339: 1608-1609.

50- Venuta A, Bertolani P, Pepe P, Francomano M, Piovano P, Ferrari P. Do pacifiers cause latex allergy? Allergy. 1999;54:1007.

51- Niggemann B, Kulig M, Bergmann R, Wahn U. Development of latex allergy in children up to 5 years of age—a retrospective analysis of risk factors. Pediatr Allergy Immunol. 1998;9:36-39.

52- Medically reviewed by Karen Gill, Written by RhonaLewis.Healthline.com. Aug 2020

53- American Academy of Pediatric Dentistry. Policy on pacifiers. The Reference Manual of Pediatric Dentistry. American Academy of Pediatric Dentistry; 2024:79-82.

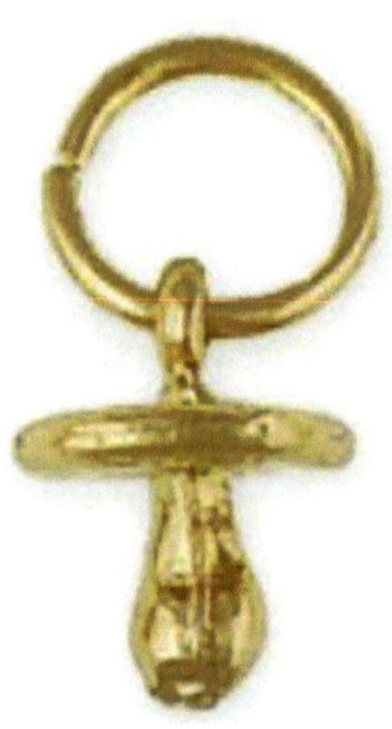

ABOUT THE AUTHOR

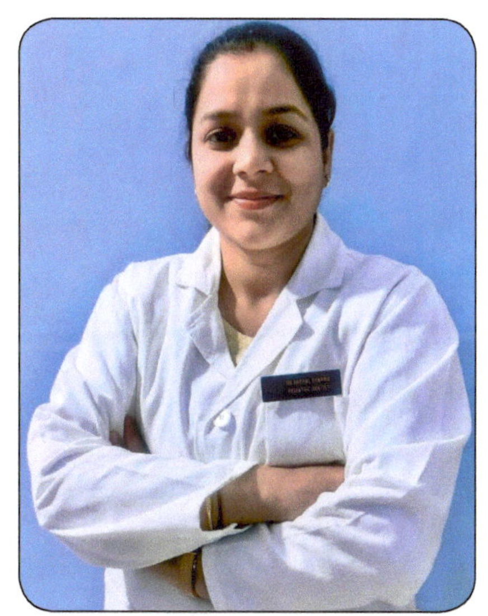

Dr. Anchal Sharma is a dedicated Pediatric dentist with over 15 years of experience in providing high-quality dental care for children of all ages. She earned her Bachelor of Dental Surgery (BDS) degree from Bharati Vidyapeeth's Dental College, Navi Mumbai. She also holds a master's degree in *Pediatric dentistry* from *ITS Dental College and Hospital*, Ghaziabad.

Dr. Anchal specializes in a wide range of pediatric dental services, including preventive care, Behaviour management, special needs dentistry, and early Orthodontic Assessment. Outside her practice, she is committed to advancing oral health education and participates in community outreach programs aimed at promoting good dental habits from an early age. She frequently partners with schools to educate children and their parents about the importance of maintaining good dental health and various effective methods to achieve it.

Dr. Anchal is an active member of *Indian Dental Association*. She also runs an Instagram channel where she shares her expert advice through easy-to-follow tutorials, myth-busting facts, and practical dental care tips to help maintain good dental health in children.

When not working, Dr. Anchal cherishes her role as a doting mother and wife and enjoys spending quality time with her family. She is an avid reader who enjoys staying informed about the latest advancements in dental technology and techniques.